To my beautiful daughters Zoe and

Jocelyn, thank you for making me smile

every day!

Forward

First of all, fellow hygienist, let me congratulate you on choosing such a great career! If you just graduated, and are anything like I was, you have spent a good deal of time wondering what the real working world is like...wishing there was a book or website that would fill you with wisdom that you did not receive in school. I too searched for that information, but came up dry! So, after 13 years of full time practice in a variety of settings, I decided to reveal my secrets to being a successful hygienist. This is the exact opposite of a clinical text book on "How to clean teeth." You better have learned that in school! Instead, it is an honest, direct, funny little gem filled with modest stories from my career to help you in yours. I do not have the typical credentials standing behind my name, but I respect the people I work with and love my patients. Most importantly, I treat them as a *whole person*, not just a mouth.

I shouldn't admit it, but I have never been a member of a hygiene society, nor have I attended more than the required amount of continuing education. Essentially, the field of dental hygiene has afforded me a decent paycheck working minimum hours, a job I literally *can't* take home at night, and little to no stress due to the improbability of finding a "ladder of success" to climb. Let's face it girls (and the one male hygienist reading this), unless we go back to dental school, our title and income are pretty fixed. That takes a lot of stress off when you're trying to balance work, home, and family.

It takes minimum effort to stay afloat in our career...but *with* a little elbow grease (and proper shoulder-fulcrum) you can truly make this an enjoyable 8 hour work-day. For those of you new to the field or just looking for a fresh new approach, I will share what works for me and how I stay positive even when I think I can't stand another minute of picking plaque off someone's teeth! I have written this in a manner that allows you to read it cover to cover while waiting for your board results, or throw it in your drawer at work and enjoy a couple of pages on your lunch-hour. It is just a reference book written by somebody who actually works in the trenches and wouldn't be qualified to write for a clinical journal or text-book; in other words, a breath of fresh air. If it sounds like I'm lecturing you or calling you out, I am...because I've been there. However, if I can prevent you from some small drama or embarrassment by sharing my stories and advice, I have accomplished my goal. I hope you enjoy it, laugh a little, and learn something. If you don't, then maybe you should write your own book!

Namaste and God Bless ~Jamie

Chapter 1

"Life is not measured by the number of breaths we take, but by the number of moments that take our breath away" ~Unknown

This is a smelly job! Not for the faint of heart. If you've just graduated, let me be the first to congratulate you and tell you that working is *nothing* like school. This is a pleasant surprise for many of you who, like me, hated school and couldn't wait to hold that scaler any darn way you pleased! But for the butt-kissers out there, get ready...no one is going to let you slide just because you babysat their kid or told them they were having a good hair day. You still need to get the medical history updated, calculus and stain off, give the typical floss lecture, schedule their next visit, and clean and set-up the room in 50 minutes or have the office manager breathing down your neck. And that doesn't take into account the sometimes 20 minute wait for the Doctor to do her one minute exam. Any amount of butt-kissing you do *should* be to the assistants, God bless them. They can be your best-friend or your worst enemy. And, let me forewarn you, they are always right and they know a whole lot more about dentistry than you do! If they ask you for help, do it with a smile and then remember to do it the next day without being asked. They work harder than anyone in the office, get paid the least, and have to deal with the Doctor's attitude one-on-one all day. They are truly saints, so give 'em the respect they deserve! Karma always comes back around, so offer to help clean up their rooms and run instruments. When you need help with a perio chart, they will be there with a smile ☺

Finding a job

So, you need a job. Where do you look? There are

almost too many options these days with the Internet and temp agencies galore. I suggest getting your resume in order, not too long and not too detailed, and drop it off at local offices. Wear something nice ("church" clothes), but NOT a suit, and walk in with a smile. Ask if the doctor is busy. If he is, introduce yourself and hand your resume to the girl behind the desk. Try to make small-talk, but avoid being chatty. Let them know in your cover letter that they can share your resume with a friend if they know someone hiring and that you will temp...and *please*, for your sake, have someone with mega grammar skills proof-read it all before you hand it out or send it anywhere. I have seen offices throw out good resumes based on poor grammar or silly typo mistakes more often than not. That is your best bet for getting work in the beginning. And be ready for that wake-up call at 5:30 am!

I started with a temp agency and it allowed me

to work in a variety of settings to see how I handled different schedules, styles, etc... I learned a lot from the other hygienists I worked with. Ask questions and use these days to expand your small amount of school knowledge because once you get a job, you may be the only hygienist there. I hate to break it to you, but very little of what you learn in school is useful when you're working. They teach you what you need to know to pass the boards, not get through an eight hour day with 13 patients who don't want to be there and don't care that they should be *wrapping* the floss around their teeth. There are days OHI and ergonomics go by the wayside just to get to the next person on the list. The longer you work, the more adept you become and soon you will be doing your patient education while you schedule their recall, buzz the Doctor and pack their goody bag. I would say it took a full one to two years of working full-time before I had the confidence that it takes to be a good hygienist. That is really all you need to succeed, a confident attitude and love for your patients.

When you get an interview, please relax! You have nothing to bring to the table at this point but a personality! Whether you just received your board's results or have been a stay-at-home mom for the past five years, you will not measure up to the other applicants that have been working. You need a positive attitude and a smile. Don't apologize for anything and remember that your pay scale will be on the low end...that is a good thing as far as the doctor is concerned. She likes the idea of paying someone less, and will often skimp on experience for a good attitude. Take whatever she offers without hesitation and then work your butt off to prove yourself over the next six months. Ask for a review and state why you think you deserve a raise based on performance and production, not because you need money to pay bills. Stay confident that you will get what you ask for and you will. Positive thinking goes a long way in this field!

With the economy like it is (and an over-saturation of new hygienists) it is more difficult than ever to find a job—including a good sub job. Here in Michigan, there is even talk of putting some hygiene programs on hold for one or two years as less than 10% of recent grads have jobs. We interview even our subs face to face, and without experience, you need a creative way to stand out in the crowd. A gal dropped off a coffee mug filled with treats and a thank you note recently, and it moved her up on our call list! ;o)

Keeping a job

When you receive that wonderful phone call asking when you can start, make it a priority to walk into work each day with a smile and try to leave your home-life and negativity in the car. Everyone at the office has their own issues going on and no one needs to be affected by your crappy morning. It's OK to joke about it once in awhile, but don't make a habit of complaining about your life at work. And certainly refrain from letting it affect the quality of your work. If you can't perform like you know is expected of you, call in sick and help find a substitute. If you have something big going on that will be a concern for a while, speak to your employer. Again, don't whine! Just inform her of your circumstances and apologize for letting it affect your work. She will likely offer help or time off instead of loosing you. Offer to find your own sub if you need a week or more off. And remember, being late (as in the patient is already sitting in your chair) more than once in a blue moon is a sure-fire way to get the axe. I've seen people be let go because of chronic tardiness, negative attitudes, know-it-all attitudes, and most recently, being too rough and hurting a patient. You may think this could never be you, but if your life is in chaos, everything else is affected as well.

I have learned this lesson the hard way. I was told by one employer many years ago that I wear my emotions on my sleeve and it is not appropriate for this line of work. I also spoke to patients about my personal life when they didn't inquire about it. I hear hygienists do this all the time. Please, for the patient's sake, do not ramble on about your weekend plans, your mom's back surgery or your husband's foul mood because the Packer's lost! It's a different story if they ask you, but avoid being Chatty Cathy to everyone. Hygienists do this because they hate silence and they want to stay on time. They leave their instruments in the patient's mouth to prevent them from responding. If you are going to speak, wipe your instrument on the 2x2 at the end of the question or statement so that your patient can respond if they wish. And, instead of chatting through the entire appointment, try asking a couple brief questions before you get started. "How was your weekend?" or "How are your kids doing?" Then look them in the eye and really listen to their answer as you lay them back. Make a note in the chart so you can remember tidbits next time.

If they take an interest in getting to know you and ask you questions, then by all means answer them. Otherwise, refrain from telling them your personal bio. Many don't care. They just want a quick, painless cleaning so that they can get on with their day. The best place to chat is while you are waiting for the Doctor to come do her exam. I always buzz when I start polishing, or grab her in the middle of my appointment if she has a lengthy appointment coming up. Keep the patient occupied so that the wait doesn't seem like an imposition.

Difficult situations

Difficult situations are definitely the best

teachers, so when you come by a tough time in your career try to look around and see what lesson you can learn instead of just complaining. If it helps, ask another staff member to have coffee with you or go online and look for hygiene chat rooms. I've never been on one, but I know they're out there. Finding someone who has experienced what you are going through helps tremendously!

I am writing this in a way that I would have devoured in my first years of practicing. I felt so lost, always the "lone" hygienist of the office. If I ran into an issue I hadn't experienced before with a patient, I had no one but the Doctor to go to. Sometimes the dentist made me feel stupid for not knowing, often because he didn't know either. Unfortunately, it is common place for an employer in any field to make their staff look dim-witted instead of admitting ignorance themselves. Don't take it personally when it happens, just keep looking elsewhere and eventually you'll find your answer. Sometimes it's when you stop looking that you find it staring you in the face. This is with life in general, so it's a good lesson to learn early on!

Knowing when to move on

The most important factor in keeping a job, in my opinion, is getting along with *everyone* in the office. That means NO gossip ladies!!! I am as guilty of it as anyone, but it is still a quick way out the door. Remember that Karma thing! If you don't like someone, avoid them, but be pleasant if you must speak to them. If you have a problem with their work or attitude, speak to them in a non-confrontational way. They may not realize they are affecting you. If you have tried to resolve something yourself and have gone through the chain of command and still do not feel things have improved, start looking for another job. You can only change yourself and *your* environment. Complaining and gossip have never changed anyone. Every negative comment you make will come back at you. It's simple law-of attraction stuff. If you haven't read *The Secret*, please head to the library pronto and save yourself a ton of headaches. Faith and positive thinking have gotten me through many unpleasant working conditions, but there may still be a time to move on.

Each time I have (reluctantly) left a position, I have found a better paying one with a more stable employer and a staff that I have more in common with. In fact, their beliefs and interests seem to parallel mine more fully each time. In my 13 year career, I have left seven different jobs for a variety of reasons, but I have never been fired or let go. I always know when it's time to move on. Once it was because I found out the dentist was guilty of billing fraud, another time it was because I found a position with better pay, and twice because of a move. Last time, I just did not feel like I "fit" with the other staff members. You learn as much as you can from one environment, then search out the next. It's a great way to keep from getting bored! Each office I've moved *up* to has been subsequently better clinically and emotionally for me, while challenging the new skills that I acquired at the prior office. Each dentist has had a better attitude and chair-side manner, and been a better clinician. Don't fight change...embrace it! It is, after all, the only thing we can truly count on in this world! (Although, Taurus' and Capricorn's are capable of a one office career!)

Chapter 2~Respect your employer

*How many hygienists does it take to change
a light bulb?
One--She stands still while the office
revolves around her.*

"It is amazing how much you can accomplish

when it doesn't matter who gets the credit."

Unknown

This is an essential principle for any team. And I'm not just talking about the people *under* you. Hygienists get the title "Prima Donna" (which *Wikipedia* defines as "the lead female singer in the opera who is typically egotistical, irritable and holds a higher opinion of herself than others do") all the time. I do not care for this personality type, hygienist or not. I have worked for and with a couple of people who fit this definition, so watch out for these traits and move on when you find them. But above all, be careful you don't fall into this category yourself. It can be quite easy to do. You are typically the highest paid employee with the most education, so why should you empty a garbage can or file charts, right? Because it helps the team, that's why! *Karma*...gonna bring it up here again!!! Try not to be the last to get to work or the first to leave. It's OK once in awhile, but not every day. If you have commitments because of your kids, try to have someone else (a husband maybe??) pick them up or drop them off one day a week so you can give other staff members a break. Bring occasional treats to the office to share. Bake, grab a dozen bagels on the way, or add a latte to your order at Starbucks because you left the assistant with a mess yesterday when you had to go to a parent-teacher meeting. Ask the receptionist if she needs anything done (she always will), and she'll be sure to tell your boss how helpful you are when review time comes up. Stress is a production killer! That is bad news for all involved, so pitch in where ever you can. Sure your instruments could use a little sharpening, but if the Doctor is 30 minutes behind, offer to deliver anesthesia, take an x-ray or clean a room. You could make a huge difference in how their day goes and that can set the tone for the rest of the week!

Respect your employer

Your boss has been through a lot to get where she is. Give them the utmost respect now and years after you've been working there. The amount of knowledge dental students must cram into their brains and the amount of emotional and personal strife they encounter while in Dental School makes what we go through look like kindergarten recess. Ask your boss about school, after a couple of stories you may look at him quite differently. We are NOT equals.

We do not endure the same amount of daily stress they do because they have to deliver both clinically and financially. They have the worry of keeping the lights on and writing our paychecks and learning the next high-tech way of doing things (and paying for it). They have ethics, liability and the guy down the street to keep up with. We just waltz in, clean teeth for eight hours and go home. If we don't make our little goal of $1000, absolutely nothing happens to us. We just come in and try again tomorrow. Some of you didn't even know you had a goal and if so, need to go to work tomorrow and ask what it is! If the Doctor doesn't hit his massive goal of $5,000 per day, he starts stressing about how to pay the bills, keep his wife's credit card paid off and put enough money into retirement so that he won't have to work until he's 70. It really adds up.

So, give him a break. It's his office and he is entitled to call the shots. Your way may have worked better for you at school or you last office, but this time it's his call. I have found that butting heads on an issue never works, but if I do what my boss wants me to for long enough to prove it isn't working; he or she at least respects me for trying. Then they ask for my opinion. Respect will go a long way here.

Teams still have one leader

An office should be looked at as a team. The coach keeps people motivated and organized, and the players work together toward a common goal. If one player is not holding up to the standards of the team, the whole is inefficient. The Doctor should be the leader...case closed. When an office manager or receptionist is given power that the Doctor should have, it complicates a whole lot of issues. It is also, at times, a sign that the Doctor is a weak or inexperienced leader. Unfortunately, I have found this to be the case more often than not. Most people do not choose to go to Dental School to run an office full of PMS-y women, they do so for the challenge of restoring teeth and creating smiles. It is rare to find an exceptional clinical dentist who is also good at running his/her practice. With that being said, it is still a good idea to treat the Doctor as the coach. They will appreciate your respect and direct you through the appropriate channels to get your needs met. Remember to do so with a smile. I tell my kids all the time "whining makes me deaf."

How to get a raise

I've already touched on this one, but I do have some suggestions here. Let me inform you that your skill level will rarely coincide with your hourly pay. A Dentist usually has a general idea what their office's hygiene production runs and has come up with a rate that they feel is appropriate. It will vary greatly. I have made between $13 and $35 an hour in my career.

Sometimes no benefits or holiday pay at all, other times full medical insurance, profit sharing, 401K, vacation/sick pay...the works. It all depends on what type of office/dentist you work for. Some put their staff's needs parallel to their own because they know that if they take care of them well, they will perform accordingly.

Others just shove as much money into their own pocket as they can and take the "dime-a-dozen" approach to hiring and keeping help. Ask about staff turn-over before you take the job. Knowing why past people left and how many hygienists have been through the doors over the past five years will keep you from making a poor decision when it comes to which position you accept. This is assuming you have more than one offer. If not, give it a try! I have learned more from the difficult experiences in my life than the easy ones.

With that said, here's what you should do when

you want to stay at an office and feel you deserve a pay increase.

1. Track hygiene production for one month. This can be done by computer or on the schedule by hand. Some offices do this anyway. Ask the receptionist for help if you need it (but don't include the Doctor's exam fee.)

2. Do a search online to see what other hygienists in your area are making. www.payscale.com is an excellent source to start with. It won't guarantee a raise, but will give you something more concrete to present than "Sarah's making more than me...whine, whine, whine." If you know other hygienist's in the immediate area you work, average out their pay and bring that to the table as well.

3. Ask the Doctor if you can speak with her at some point "this week." That tells her it isn't urgent and allows her to fit you in where she

can give you her full attention.

4. Present your case in a clear, concise manner and stay calm. I've left many reviews in tears only to find out they gave me the raise anyway! Just because your boss wants to point out some areas you need to work on does not mean you're an awful hygienist or that your performance is terrible, it just means that--big surprise--you're not *perfect.* Take notes and really act interested in what suggestions they have, even if you're not! They often forget about them the next week anyway, but it makes them feel validated when you *listen* to them. Pick one area they said you needed work on and do some reading/research. Maybe there is something to learn that could make your day go smoother after all!

5. *BELIEVE YOU WILL GET THE RAISE*. That is the

most important, often overlooked component. If you just complain to your husband all the time that you'll "never be paid what you're worth", then you never will!

Chapter 3~The Staff

"Good friends are truly the spice of life"

Appreciate the Assistants

The most integral component to success in a dental office is a good assistant. They usually run the place. I have never understood why they aren't paid their weight in gold, but I've never run a practice either. They are almost always intelligent and talented enough to have made it through dental school, but finances or life circumstances kept them from realizing it. If there is one thing you can do in your career that matters, build a friendship with them. Help them. They are some of the most giving, hard-working, multi-talented people you will meet. Unfortunately, they can be easily taken advantage of by others for that very reason. Be sure you are not one of those people.

I have encouraged some of my assistant friends to move on to better-suited careers, just by telling them how amazing they are. They sometimes have self-esteem barriers preventing them from seeing their true potential. No one has ever told them they can be anything they dream, and they may have a million excuses when you tell them. Regardless, your life will be enriched by spending time outside of the office with them. The friendships I've made have turned out, at times, to be the purpose of my being at an office in the first place. Thinking of them will always bring a smile to my face for many years to come. They are genuinely good people and I am blessed to have had them in my life...many of them still are!

Do your share, and then some

I've already touched on this subject, but the most important thing you can do in the staff's eyes is to go above and beyond what is expected of you. Your employer will likely be thrilled if you come to work on time, hit your production goal once in awhile and cause as little tissue trauma as possible. After a couple of years at this, it becomes very easy to grow complacent, bored and lazy, headed toward burn-out. Most offices have either the back or front well-ran, but rarely both. There is usually one area where another person needs to be hired, but isn't. Become that person. Make the most of your day by looking around for things you know how to do. Offer to learn something new. I have done my own billing, tracked production, answered the phone, worked on collections, managed recall, called insurance companies, caught up sterilization, remade and re-cemented temporaries, helped with ortho, taken impressions (poorly), cleaned the office, re-taped instruments, filed and pulled charts, made up new patient charts, organized the dungeon (better known as the basement), done laundry, reorganized cabinets, etc... There is *always* something out of the normal scaling and polishing to do if you look hard enough. I was told recently that I'm too valuable to file charts, so now I only do it when he's not looking! :o)

Social Gatherings

The best way to keep a large (or small) office running smoothly is to have social get-togethers outside the office. This can include meeting for a drink after work, a BBQ at someone's house, a scrap-booking or jewelry party, or just going to a seminar together. If your office doesn't already do this, it may be because no one wants to take the time to organize it. The larger the office, the more difficult it is to get everyone involved. Try suggesting it at the next office meeting. The more you do it, the more fun it is. People are so different when you get to know them as their real self. You may even find that someone you are regularly irritated with is a kick in the pants after hours! Do this as often as possible and your work day goes by so fast because you feel like you work with your friends, and you do!

Emptying your own garbage can

If you dare skip over this section you might as well put the book down now! *Please*...do not...ever...expect anyone else to empty your garbage can. Even if the office has cleaning people, you throw your bloody 2x2's and saliva strewn fluoride trays in there all day and should try to keep it from overflowing all over the inside of your cabinet. It's even OK to empty it in the middle of the day if it's full! It's even OK to go around the office and empty the rest of the garbage cans!!! I know, you never thought much about it. That's why I'm writing this book.

Chapter 4~The Patient

"A patient is not an interruption of our work;

he is the purpose of it"

~Unknown

The most important person in any office should be the patient. They are the reason you have a job and the person who actually makes sure you get a paycheck. Without that person sitting in your chair, you would not be making a living. Remember this every day! No matter how rude, quiet, grungy or wonderful your patient is, they are the purpose of your work, not an interruption of it. I know how good that coffee smells that the receptionist just made, but you cannot pretend that you didn't notice your patient was due for bitewings so that you have an extra ten minutes between patients. I've been there, and I *have* done that...more times than I should admit. I am writing this book from an honest, straight-forward perspective. I know you will encounter these situations because I have. And I have at times made the wrong choice and regretted it later. If I can at least give you a head's up on what is to come, you will hopefully be better prepared to make better choices than I was.

Treating the whole patient,

not just their mouth

We learned a lot about the human body in hygiene school. Remember those hours with the smelly dead people they made us dissect? Your patient is more than a mouth, so if they sit down with that sigh that says, "I just want to get this over with," get your brain motoring and let the fuses connect. Do they seem stressed or depressed? Are they overweight? Is there a family history of diabetes? Are they clenching or grinding? Which hand is their dominant hand? Do they have full use of it? These are not things that you find on their medical history, so always be on your toes. When you see signs of perio in a patient that has excellent oral hygiene, your sirens should be going off saying,"something else is going on here!"

Let's discuss the bruxors. I have found that "white collar" areas have the same incidence of perio as the "blue collar" offices and that in the higher socio-economic patients, perio problems are mostly caused by stress and occlusal problems, not bacteria! Look for signs by watching them swallow while looking at their face. Are their masseter muscles over- developed? Do they have a square, tight jaw line? Are their teeth short or flattened? Do they have severe recession or abfractions without the presence of inflammation? These are all important signs to document, as your patient is likely to state they do not clench the first time you discuss it with them.

Explain what clenching is to your patient—simply touching their teeth together when they are not eating or speaking. Tell them to pay attention when they drive, check their e-mail, weight-lift, sleep, etc... Tell them not to chew gum (Some people get addicted and it is a form of bruxing, causing the muscle memory of clenching). Your patient may come back six months later and say, "You were so right, I *do* clench!" If your employer isn't aware of the correlation between perio and clenching, find some literature and bring it to his attention. Find a seminar on bruxism and occlusal therapy you can attend together. Night time bite splints are an integral part of my current office's perio therapy and should be addressed at your office as well.

*** I had the pleasure and privilege to have Dr. Major Ash as one of my patients years ago. Anyone who knows anything about occlusion has heard his name and likely read one or two of his text-books. I actually worked for his daughter in Ann Arbor. Dr. Carolyn Ash, was the first licensed female Prosthodontist in the state of California. Working with this family of dentists (one brother is an Endodontist and the other is an Orthodontist) helped me gain a new respect for how all the specialties complement each other and work toward a common goal. I also gained an interest in occlusion and full-mouth restoration as a result. The two years I spent there were invaluable to my career and added depth to my treatment practices that wouldn't have been possible without them. I deeply appreciate their brilliance and would like to thank them for accepting me as a member of their dental family, even though it was for a short time.

OHI—How to stop bugging your patients to floss

One of the most common things I hear in a day

is, "Thank you for not lecturing me on flossing." Patients really do learn to tune out the routine lecture we learned in school. They tell me the "last girl" was rough, talked incessantly, or worse...had no personality. Find a fresh approach to OHI. Instead of asking *if* they are flossing, try asking how often they floss. They will usually answer "not enough" with a tone of complete guilt. I prefer "Are you flossing daily, or near to it?" That gives me a clear yes or no and I let them talk after instead of me. It saves the lecture. If they aren't flossing, I ask them if they have trouble doing it or remembering...in a concerned manner. If they don't remember, have them leave it out somewhere like near the TV, computer or in their car. If it's been in the bathroom drawer for 45 years and they haven't noticed it, why would they see it now? If they have trouble, I ask them if they'd like to watch me floss their teeth. Most say "Yes, that would help!" and we find out together that they have a technique issue standing in the way of victorious flossing. Floss-picks and stimudents are a good alternative if their pockets are within normal limits, but if they have any 5mm or above, they won't be effective in those areas.

If they have trouble (Men, people with arthritis, small mouths, etc), then I immediately say "Let me give you some other aides that might be easier for you." Their faces light up!!! "You mean, I don't have to floss?" their eyes seem to say. I am a HUGE fan of Butler GUM Go-Betweens or any proxabrush. I wish I would've invented them! They are so small they fit almost anywhere with a millimeter of tissue loss, and they are better stimulators than floss. Get the mirror out if they seem interested and demonstrate where and how to use them. Between 2/3 and 14/15 seem to be problem areas for most people to keep clean and they are easy to maneuver there. I tell them to go through their mouth and see where it fits. If it doesn't fit there, then they don't need it...floss is enough (see, I do still get that in!) I also tell them to use it after they brush so they can see what is left between their teeth when they only brush and that it is more important *that* they clean inter- proximally, than *how*.   Use a cross-section picture of the periodontium or a plastic model and show them where gum disease lives...that they can't see it or feel it till too much destruction has occurred. So many patients tell me that they've never been told *why* to floss, just hounded about doing it. I prefer to do OHI at the end of the appointment, that way I've gained their trust and friendship by hearing about their family and answering their questions first. Once they know that I am trying to spare them thousands of dollars in perio treatment, I never have to lecture again!

Life Coaching, Astrology and other
tidbits I'd like to share

This is a section devoted to what I've enjoyed most about my career...getting to know my patients. When you are within one inch of someone's personal space for one hour every 6 months, you can get either really uncomfortable, or really educated about the human race. Each person is so different and really needs an original approach to get through to them. So, where do you start? Deciding if they are Type A or Type B is a good place. The A's like a lot of information and will ask many questions, I typically write things down for them to check out at the stores or online. The B's just want to relax...so give them that. Save most of your communication for when you start polishing and filter your words to the important ones. They don't want to hear about you or your life and they don't want to tell you about theirs. Be specific about what you'd like them to do. Not just

"You need to floss more!", but "Mr. Jones, you should try to floss more because you have inflammation around your molars and if you don't, I'm afraid you will need Gum Disease treatment soon. I'd like to see you in 4 months instead of 6 to make sure we are doing enough." And that's ALL you say, period! If they say OK, then schedule a 4 month recall. If they say nothing back, schedule the regular 6 month interval and document in the chart that you suggested a 4 month recall and they declined it. Get a decline form typed up for them to sign if you don't already have one.

You don't need a 6 hour CE class with an overly excited speaker who had one too many sugar-free Red Bulls to tell you that! It's not complicated. You may have touched a nerve, but they don't want you to know quite yet. They may come back in 6 months and say "What you said last time really got to me, I floss nightly now."

ALL patients like to hear that it's not fully their fault. Find something else to put partial blame on. Genetics, health, stress, hormones, dexterity, etc... They need to feel like you are their *partner* in this battle, not their *mother*. They will respect you more if you are honest and straightforward, but need to see a certain tenderness to trust you. That being said, you can't change everyone. Know who to save your breath on and notate it in the chart as "uninterested in OHI." Make them sign a Periodontal Treatment Decline sheet. That alone will often make them reconsider their attitude and start asking the appropriate questions to remove their fear.

I use Astrology to decide how to approach my patients in the most effective manner. I know, many of you are afraid to keep reading now, wondering if this is some crazy "New Age" book, but I promise you that this is the extent of it. I've been studying true astrology for almost 10 years. Not the blurb you read in the paper about what will happen to you today, but what personality strengths or weaknesses people are born with. My friend and colleague Jessica told me to toot my own horn here, as I am quite accurate, but it's not rocket science. It is a little more detailed than the Type A or B approach. For those of you not comfortable, skip ahead. For the others, I'll give you a quick guide to turn to the next time you have a patient you can't figure out:

Pisces (February 20-March 20) Answer their questions; they like to hear about you.

Virgo (August 22-September 23) Very inquisitive; hit the "health" aspect hard.

Aries (March 21-April 20) Be quick, and talk while you work, they don't sit still for long.

Taurus (April 21-May 21) Are more concerned with how their teeth look than how healthy they are. Discuss whitening, veneers or Invisaliagn.

Gemini (May 22-June 21) and Sagittarius (November 23-December 22) Have fun with them and stay positive, tell them what they are doing right, ask them about their travels.

Cancer (June 22-July 22) Wants to find a personal connection with you, may be withdrawn at first.

Leo (July 23-August 21) Find something to complement them on, talk sports or kids.

Scorpio (October 24-November 22) and Capricorn (December 23-January 20) Money talks with them, find a way to decrease their out of pocket expense ("By crowning this tooth before it hurts, we should be able to prevent a root canal in the future which would be an additional $800.").

Aquarius (January 21-February 20) and Libra (September 24-October 23) Typically artsy, find an original approach as unique as they are by asking them what they do for a living first.

I also do a little Life Coaching on the side, and tend to offer advice to patients on a daily basis. Hygienists are much like hairdressers or bartenders. People feel comfortable opening up to us because they trust us. And the prone position doesn't hurt either. I've suggested people quit jobs, change careers, go back to work, find a hobby, reconnect with a child, the list goes on. And why not? If we aren't on this earth to help inspire each other to find our life's purpose and live to our highest potential, then why bother? God may have made me good at scraping junk off people's teeth, but I believe he made me a hygienist mostly because I could connect with the people that needed me in some way. Stay open during your day and you'll be pleasantly surprised by the ways God will use you. The people I work with are often amazed that I "got through that guy" or had so much in common with someone or was able to network in multiple ways during an appointment. I often ask for a patient's card or give them mine. You can have some funky ones printed up easily with www.vistaprint.com. Use them for personal reasons, business or pleasure. The main point of this section is: make the most out of your day, and the rewards are endless

Chapter 5~Your Perio Program

"Excellence is a habit" ~Esther Wilkins, RDH, DMD

Own it!

What does that mean exactly? We were taught in school to help the patient take ownership of his or her condition, right? Well, guess who's responsible for making sure the patient is educated fully? If you are the "solo" hygienist in the office, this responsibility will likely fall on you. If there is a team of you, you should already have something in place so that the entire office is handling perio the same. It doesn't matter so much *how* you do things, but that you are sticking to some type of protocol, and I hate protocol! But in this case, it is important. Most dentists have totally different opinions about when and how to treat perio. If you've never sat down and discussed what your employer would like done, you may need to approach her yourself, and please do so ASAP! Making perio an integral part of your office can literally double hygiene production, plus the obvious benefit to the patients' overall health.

I find the older the dentist, the more difficult it is to get her on board when it comes to bringing perio up with patients of record. However, they rarely have trouble when a new patient comes in after a 15 year absence. Having walls of calculus to remove that the patient can see and feel make light work of getting a root planing scheduled. But what about the patient that has been faithful about their recall for 15 years and flosses and lives next door to your boss? I have seen 8mm pockets and exudate that the dentist turns a blind eye to for fear of losing them as a patient and/or friend. The dentist will sometimes feel neglectful for missing it and will ignore it, or tell you to just "get down there and clean it out" during a routine prophy. I urge you—*please*, don't do it because you're not doing anyone any favors! This will happen to you during your career if it hasn't already. You have two choices when it does. You can either do it and inform the patient that there is gum disease present and Dr. X wants to be conservative for now (start looking for another job), or refuse (not in front of the patient) and immediately ask for a meeting to discuss how to handle future issues. Once your employer understands that you are capable of running a successful perio program and not everyone will need thousands of dollars in perio surgery, he may be more open to your suggestions.

Where to start

Like I said before, if nothing is in place or written down, ask your boss or office manager if a meeting can be scheduled. There are also many wonderfully informative seminars on perio that the whole office can attend so that everyone knows what to say, how to bill, and how to handle insurance questions. Consistency is the key and the fluidity with which the staff describes the procedure is what makes the patient think your office has it together.

Would you rather go to a medical office that is brand new and fancy, but the staff never seems to know what's what, or a slightly old, out of date one that runs like clockwork? No brainer right? Some offices hire a consultant to come in and train the staff, but I find that approach flat and predictable with little room for the hygienist to individualize care based on patient need. It's usually more about the bottom line when an office hires a consulting firm. Basically, they don't want *your* opinion; they just want to "Stepfordize" the practice while increasing revenue. Most employers spend more than they make with this approach, so if you can talk your boss into letting you try your way it's going to save money.

What you need

- At least 2 very sharp perio set ups with all the posterior graceys (9-10 total scalers). And don't sharpen unless they need it! I mark a dull set up with colored tape when it's dirty, then once it's sterilized I go through to see which ones actually need sharpening, then sterilize it again. It's not necessary to sharpen every instrument every day. Get your daily stress relief from yoga or running, don't take it out on your instruments!

- An ultrasonic scaler that can hold Chlorhexidine and has a slim tip is also a must. There is much controversy on how to use this, but I like to use it at the end. You DO NOT remove calculus with a slim tip; you use one of the shorter, wide-tipped inserts for that. I find I don't have as much tactile sensitivity with it, so if I use my hands first I typically know where I need to do extra work at the end. But always go through the whole mouth with it, not just the deep pockets. The other reason I like to use it last is that I rinse often during the appointment, so it's a final lavage that removes left-over debris and more bio-film than hand scaling. Current evidence supports the theory that hand scaling removes a precious cell-activating protein layer, so again, use it for the fine scaling if nothing else. We no longer need to remove an entire layer of cementum to be effective like once thought. I graduated long enough ago to have done that for years, so old dogs can learn new tricks!

- You also need a perio chart that is easy to

record on and use. When it's 2010 and I flip back in the chart and see the last scribbling was 2006, we have a problem and the perio chart takes top priority over all else. Recording furcations, mobility and recession is a must. I've fallen into the habit of only recording pockets of 4mm and up in stable patients. So far, it's working OK, but it's probably not ideal. A full perio chart of all pockets every six months is just overkill to me. It makes the patient dread coming in. Not that I think we should skip probing though. I do probe at every visit, but if nothing has changed, then why write it all down. It's a quick way to burn out. Do a full one every 1-1/2 years if the patient is flossing and stable. For a new patient, make it as detailed and colorful as you possibly can and use it for patient education as well. Healthy patients deserve to hear about their *lack* of periodontal disease as much as the unhealthy ones.

- Perio forms are needed to educate the patient about what procedures they are having or had done and for the purpose of declining treatment. We use a similar one to the X-ray decline form that most offices have. I have them sign it even if they want to go on a 6 month recall when I suggested a 4 month, or if they "just want a regular cleaning" when they should be receiving a perio prophy (4910). You can't be too careful when it comes to covering your butt and your boss' too! Besides, we all know that the people who don't continue with the soft tissue maintenance program often need re-treatment anyway. Wait until they return to their pre-root planing state and then you can say "I tried to tell you!" Few patients fall off the wagon twice.

- Also, a video, pamphlet and/or model are helpful during the education phase. It is important to their continuing health that they understand what they are having done and why they need it so that the process can be halted. Each patient will respond to a different approach, so have a wide variety of materials on hand.

- Last but not least is proper billing. Be sure to answer any of the patients or receptionist's questions about fees, insurance or billing codes. 4341 for an entire quad, 4342 for 1-3 teeth. If you don't know, go online or attend a seminar. Fees should not be a surprise when patients get to the end of their appointment. Make sure it is discussed before they schedule.

- Optional items are power toothbrushes, waterpiks, prescription fluoride, mouthwash, and MI Paste to include in the program or sell. Somehow, handing the patient a $100 sonic toothbrush that the office paid $50 for makes them feel better about spending $1000 on their gums. Go figure :o)

What to do when you get bored

Well, this will ultimately decide how long you practice...if you can keep your back and neck "in line" that is. Once you've been at an office long enough, and you have your own patients that are faithful about returning regularly, you find out that you either like a clean mouth, or you don't. Those that enjoy picking at clean lower anteriors for 15 minutes while getting their patients latest teen daughter drama will be able to stay for many years at one practice. It becomes more about the patient for them, and they shiver at the memory of the two appointment debridement's they did in the beginning of their career because the patients were so uneducated and overdue. For these hygienists, a patient with little debris is a reward for all the hard work they did when they first started.

For me, however, I can only do one or two of these people in a day without wanting to yell,"Where's the good stuff?" I actually *enjoy* calculus removal...I guess you could say I even get off on it. Crazy, I know, but I suspect there are more like me out there. If I get through the whole mouth with only my 204-S, and am left with an empty 2x2, I feel NO sense of satisfaction. It's selfish to think that I enjoy when people are unhealthy, but I think it's more about the fact that I get to help them get healthy. I look at it as an artist would. I love that I get to finish a masterpiece every 60 minutes many times a day. There is so much gratification to me when I see them lick the back of their teeth and say "Ahhhh, thank you!"

So, if you are one of the few hygienists that have 90% of your patients healthy and stable like I do, what do you do when you get bored? Well, the cure for that is to look for "spots" to treat, like a 5mm pocket that bleeds on the distal of #3 that's been there for the last three appointments. Have them come back for a 30 minute appointment, numb them, root plane the entire area around #2 and 3, and bill out as code 4342. We call it a "mini-quad", but the ADA code states that it is for one to three teeth. It is also an excellent way to ease a lifetime 6 month adult prophy patient into perio treatment. Once they see that it doesn't hurt and wasn't a big deal, they may be more likely to have other areas treated. (I know the new grads covered these codes in school, but wanted to include it for those that have been practicing for years and did not.)

If a patient of record comes in regularly and only has pockets of 5mm and over in the posterior, with no bleeding in the anterior, why should they have their entire mouth done? Some patients will say no to full mouth scaling and root planing, but yes to "just the back." They know they don't get back there as well and can see the bleeding themselves. I often bill out the 4342 code four times and just do the molars. It's less expensive (charge half to two-thirds the cost of one quad) and it's a good way to ease them into perio treatment as well. Once they find out that it doesn't hurt, and are able to see the improvement six weeks later, they might finally be fully "on board" with you. Most insurance companies cover a 4910 if two quads have had any perio treatment at all—including the "mini-quad" code.

What I do

1. **Perio Chart ~** A new patient needs a full, detailed one. Ask many questions, highlight anything above a 4, and write important info on the chart such as: Smokes 2 packs a day, Type II Diabetic, Past Perio Surgery, etc... Put a Case Type on the top and circle or highlight it. Sit the patient up and explain it to them. Ask if they have any questions. I always explain what the classifications mean. I say "Type I is a teenager who doesn't floss, but has no tissue or bone loss, Type V needs full dentures, you are in the middle as a Type III." That gets to them...like the stages of cancer or some other disease they've heard about. It implies a more serious issue than the word

"perio." You can also say that "Type IV's usually loose one or more of their teeth, and if we don't treat this now, you are headed there quickly. It takes a long time to cause a one millimeter of bone loss, but once those bacteria live where you can't reach them, the process goes much quicker. Floss only gets 4mm under the gum line, even if you're awesome at it!" This is also the appropriate time for the health correlation speech that you perfected in school. Most offices are now charging based on Case Type, but some still just charge by the quadrant. It is best if the person in charge of billing speaks with them about cost and insurance, but if you are comfortable doing it, go for it!

***In my current office, new patients see the Doctor for an FMX and full initial exam before me. This is the way it should be done, legally speaking. He Case Types based on a little probing, looking at the bone level on the radiographs and amount of calculus present. The first time I see the patient is for scaling and root planing and they are typically under conscious sedation. I have little to no say in who needs it or what their Case Type is. I do my charting after I numb them (or at the end if there is too much calculus and I feel I won't get true readings). This is the first office I have not been the main "diagnostic gatherer" at. I don't always agree with his decision, so this is an example of how we compromise. Sometimes I talk to him about my opinion after the appointment and we change the case type. Even though his way of diagnosing isn't what I'm familiar with, it's how he's done it for years--and has a large practice of healthy patients--so who am I to argue?

2. **Perio Waiver** ~ Have them sign one if they decline perio treatment or anything perio related that you suggested. Some offices have everyone sign one to prove that they informed them which stage they were at. This really is a good idea, especially in large offices where patients see multiple hygienists. One should be on file near the perio chart. If they don't want treatment, ask them if they would like you to keep checking (by probing) for areas that get worse. They may want you to just shut up and clean their teeth and never talk about it again. As long as they signed a waiver, leave them alone. They will respect you for it and at least future appointments will be more tolerable. They may even thank you for not bugging them

about it and ask you to explain it again the next time they come in.

3. **The Root Planing (also now known as Root Debridement) appointment** ~ You don't need instruction on "how" to do this, but please make sure your instruments are sharp. And when delivering anesthesia, I now infiltrate even the mandibular thanks to Dr. Erdman. I didn't believe this was possible, but with Articaine it works great! I use less anesthesia and the patient goes through less trauma during numbing. This method is also ideal when you are "spot root planing." We use Nitrous Oxide for the majority of perio treatment and offer sedation when the patient wants their entire mouth done in one appointment. This is typically done when it has been a number of years since they were

in, or are fearful. We have them take one Xanax before bed, and another in the morning when they wake up. We schedule them first and make sure someone drops them off and picks them up. They talk during the appointment, but rarely remember a thing! It is truly a blessing for these people! We charge an extra fee because they are more difficult to work on, and ask for pre-payment. This is my favorite part of what I currently do. The transformation of their mouth in 3-4 hours is like a miracle to them. And not remembering it is all the better! This is a very rewarding way to handle perio. My boss, Dr. E, uses it the same way. He has done as many as 17 composites in one appointment! Talk about instant gratification, for both the clinician and the patient! I rarely do multiple appointment root planning now.

4. **OHI** ~ This can be done at the last RP appointment, or if the patient was sedated like mine often are, I have them come back in one week. Make it 20-30 minutes and very hands on. Use the mirror or models and give them as many "gadgets" as you think it will take to find one they will actually use. I give them an electric toothbrush at this appointment as well. Ask them how they feel the last appointment went. It will give you a sense of their attitude toward you and the office.

5. **6 week check** ~ This is the most important step in their continued progress. If they skip this, they probably think you "took care of things" and are already back to their old ways. You may not see them again till they have a toothache, but you should still call and

bug them about getting back in. This is where you will determine how much they've healed based on new probe readings. Change their recall to three or four months in the computer and notate it on the chart as well. We use PP3 or PP4 to denote perio prophy every three or four months so that everyone in the office knows what type of recall they are on. AP6 would be a regular adult prophy at a six month interval. If they, by chance, have no bleeding, then you can add the word maintenance or "maint" to their Case Type. It tells everyone that they are stable. Record what their home care routine is and give them pointers on any areas that still need attention. This is where you would decide to refer someone to a Periodontist if they still have areas that are still 6mm or above with bleeding or exudate present. I would keep a patient with a couple of 6mm pockets for at least one more recall. Sometimes 6 weeks isn't enough healing time, especially if they have other factors at play. Diabetics, clenchers, and people in need of restorative work will need more time before you make that decision.

6. **Place Perio Chip or other Antimicrobial ~** When a pocket ABOVE 5mm remains at this appointment, or exudate is present, I place a Perio Chip. (www.periochip.com) Any local antibiotic or antimicrobial should help, but I have found these chips to be easy to place, comfortable to the patient and reliable for a 1-2mm pocket reduction. This is only *after* root planing though. They have also never failed me for halting exudate. They are expensive (I've seen charges of $75-125 for each one) and insurance won't always pay for

them, but as a last resort to a specialist referral, most people say "go for it!" I think a box of 20 cost us around $400, so $20 each. If you place one, reserve it for someone with only one or two trouble spots and have them come back in six weeks for 10 minutes to re-probe there. I give a guarantee, if there is no improvement after six weeks; they get a credit on their account. I've only had this happen once since I started placing these four years ago and it was because the woman had such severe xerostomia that she didn't have enough saliva to dissolve it. Oral antibiotics can be used as well, but the only one I've found especially effective is metronidazole (Flagel). Your patient will likely vomit if they drink any alcohol while on the 10 day dosage, so you may be limited by who will be willing to go that long without a glass of Merlot.

7. **Soft Tissue Maintenance (4910)** ~ At the end of the six week check, the Doctor and I discuss the patient's recall interval, which always starts at three months. Then I make their next appointment and reiterate that they will return to their previous condition if they don't keep it. Once they are completely stable (which typically takes one year), and have little to remove, I often move them to four months. Not all offices would think this a wise move, but I have found that people are more likely to make a 4 month appointment, whereas they miss or reschedule a 3 month appointment much more. Anyone with a history of perio treatment should be on a 4910 for the rest of their life. Explain to them that gum disease doesn't "come and go", but is more like diabetes...and floss is their

insulin! If they request to go back to a 6 month recall and you feel they will be ok there, still bill with this code. And don't forget to have them sign the waiver!

8. **Change it up when it isn't working ~** Never feel like there isn't room for improvement. And do not repeat what does not work! Read journals, talk to other hygienists, brainstorm with the entire staff at the office meeting. But most of all use your intuition with each and every patient to tailor a program to meet their needs accordingly. Don't go all cookie cutter when it comes to your patients oral health...the more enthusiasm you put in, the more they get out.

Chapter 6~Ergonomics and Keeping Fit

"Never bend your head, hold it high, look the world straight in the eye"

~Helen Keller

Posture~Yikes!

This will be a short chapter because this is the one area I still struggle with. I can tell you that a little yoga can go a long way in reversing the damage we do to ourselves trying to see the lingual of #11 better. I still giggle to myself each time a patient or coworker tells me I'm a great hygienist because I spent so much time in remediation during my days at Ferris State University. Each time I had a clinical exam, I was told that I would be proficient at removing debris (which was typically invisible on a plastic tooth) with little tissue trauma, but needed to hold my instruments the way they told me and sit properly or I was going to have a short career due to body break-down. Well, somehow, they were wrong! I have only had trouble with my hands when I was pregnant and swollen. I immediately started using my own techniques and grips upon graduation and haven't gone back since! One instructor told me to do myself a favor and only work four days a week, spending the last day in the gym. I've always been active and currently teach Zumba and take Salsa lessons. Find what you love to do and it won't feel like exercise. I could tell you to sit up straight here, but instead I'll tell you to stretch after work (those big exercise balls are great for your back) and take a brisk walk on your lunch hour. These two things will help you just as much as good posture.

Loops, Ultrasonic Scalers and Sharpening

I wish I could give you great advice on magnifying eye wear, but I've never been privileged enough to own or use them. Most good cosmetic dentists would call in sick if they lost theirs, so I assume they pretty much rock! I've worked so many years *up close* to the mouth, that I would likely have a harder time getting used to them than someone new to the profession. Besides, what we do is dependent on *feel* rather than sight anyway, so it's up to you if you have an extra $1000 burning a hole in your pocket. I'd take that money and build a home gym...just sayin'.

Ultrasonic scalers and the like are invaluable to our profession. They do something our hands just can't do. However, those of you using it for every Tom, Dick and Harry regardless of how much calculus or inflammation they have should rethink your approach. Our hands have something the machines don't...and that is tactile sensitivity. I believe that while both techniques do an equal job at cleansing the tooth and stimulating the tissue, neither should be used exclusively, but rather selectively. Anyone who has worked with me is yelling right now because they know that I am an advocate of good old-fashioned hand scaling. Call me old school, go ahead. But let me explain that this is what works best, for me. I've tried using my Piezon for all adult patients, but I'm not as good at it. It takes me longer, is messier and most patients don't like it as much. Now, with that being said, I also pride myself on being one of the most gentle, yet thorough hygienists on the block. I feel more connected to the tooth and the patient without all that electricity in the way, but some of you may feel just the opposite.

What I would like to warn you about is your curette skills getting rusty. The patients that have asked me to use it have often informed me that the "last girl" didn't use those sharp, poky things at all.

And guess what? I found a whole lot of burnished, sub-gingival, left over calculus on those patients. In fact, through the years whenever I've found repeated burnished calculus on a patient, I've gone ahead and asked them how much hand scaling was typically done on them. "Very little" was always their reply. Or, "She liked that machine thing better", or "She just talked a lot." So, to conclude this ever-controversial topic, do I think every office should have an Ultrasonic Scaler? Yes, one in each hygiene operatory in fact. But, if you have been trained to use it on all adults, please spend *equal* time with your trusty 204-S. Use it at the end and do an exploratory stroke with it. Since you can go through the entire mouth, supra and sub with this specific instrument, it won't take you long. And *always* use the Ultrasonic, with antimicrobial, for perio treatment.

Ok, on to sharpening. Let me begin by saying that I am as guilty as the next girl for burnishing calculus. Any hygienist that has taken over after I've left has surely shaken her head a time or two at my demise. The point is we *all* leave calculus behind. And while none of us is perfect, we can still try to get darn close and feel happy with ourselves at the end of the day. I touched on this earlier in Chapter 5 and would like to reiterate it here as part of how to prevent body breakdown and fatigue. There are many schools of thought on sharpening, so I'll tell you what works for me. Devise a system of marking a set up (colored tape on cassette, writing "dull" on bag, etc...) that you have given a beating to with Mr. Periobreath. It's usually going to be dirty, so please only sharpen *after* they've been sterilized (if there is a way to give each hygienist her own set-ups to be responsible for, even better). Be careful though that you don't over sharpen. Wailing on all your instruments daily is going to cause thin, easy to break tips and your boss isn't going to like the replacement bill either. I suggest re-tipping. It is such a rush to get those puppies back in the mail, feels like Christmas.

I will have 10 or so instruments re-tipped every two to three months. That way, I always have my favorites, or at least one set-up super sharp. We also have purchased one of those machines so that supposedly everyone in the office can sharpen exactly the same...but they don't. It does work well after re-tipping though, because it takes off minimal edge. Again, many employers have rushed into the sterilization room to ask me what that horrible sound was. That tells me that many of you should spend less time flipping through People and more time annoying the staff!

Yoga for the RDH

If you are new to yoga, or afraid to make a fool of yourself attending a class, I'd like to give you a couple of poses to try at home. Once you're comfortable, try buying a full video or catching a class with a friend. If you don't care for it at first, try a different instructor. Most gyms have a stripped down beginner style if you are nervous about looking silly. Yoga is meant to do daily, like taking your vitamins. These can be done upon rising, during your lunch break or at night to relax before bed. I used to squeeze in some squats or a yoga pose while developing bitewings—those tiny darkrooms make you get really creative! In fact, I blame digital radiographs for the five pounds I've gained over the past year! My sister, Lisa, always says "Just do one stretch...and before you know it 15 minutes have gone by because it feels so good you just keep going." The cool thing about yoga is that it feels too easy to be called exercise. Even the least fit can do it. The benefit is that it gets to some of those small stabilizer muscles you don't use every day and the stress relieving aspect makes you so balanced and happy so that you actually feel like being active. You start to learn the value in it. The older I get, the more I learn that physical activity should be done because of the way it makes you feel, not the way it makes you look. We're never happy with that aspect anyway. If God wanted you to be a supermodel instead of a hygienist you wouldn't be reading this book! You can look these up in a yoga book or online.

Yoga Poses

Namaste

Sun Salutation

Tree

Warrior I and II

Triangle

Childs Pose

Cat and Cow

Chapter 7~Community Service

"Generosity is giving more than you can, and

pride is taking

less than you need"

~Kahlil Gibran

How to find places to volunteer

This is the single most rewarding part of what we do; help the less fortunate smile for at no charge just because we can. If you haven't done this yet, then put down this book and go Google "dental volunteers + your city and state" ASAP! An excellent site is www.dentalvolunteer.com. Ask around if anyone knows of a free clinic nearby. Call them and find out if they'll take you for just one day. You may say "Well, I'm glad I got that out of the way," or you may become a regular there. And don't give me the excuse that you're too busy. If you have even one day off per week and have golfed or read a smut magazine on that day off, *ever*, then you do have time. If you are already an active volunteer in other areas of your life, like your church or for Big Brother/Big Sister, then I'll lay off of you. This goes as well for any dentists that may be reading this. Writing off your neighbors crown doesn't count either. I know it is an act of goodwill, but come on, they could've made payments. Poor 9 year old Johnny Pop-Mouth has never seen a dentist or been told he shouldn't carry a generic 2 liter around with him and sip on it all day. Don't think it is someone else's calling...it's *all* of our calling. Remember karma here as well, it always comes back.

School Programs and Sealant Clinics

Another way of using your gifts outside of your office is to call up your local elementary school and see if you can give a talk during Children's Dental

Health Month in February. It's pretty easy to contact the ADA and get supplies, pictures to color, etc...Your employer or local dentists will often donate toothbrushes, especially if their name and contact info is printed on them (free advertising). I go in for 15 minutes and talk, answer questions and give out goodies. It's what you did for school in Community Dental Health class, no biggie. It's worth the drive there just to see the smiles on their faces when you tell them chocolate is better for their teeth than soda pop. They go home and tell their parents, "The tooth fairy told us to eat more chocolate!" ...Priceless.

If you live in or near an underprivileged community you can also talk to local dentists about starting a sealant program. I've helped out with one and basically you seal all the second graders first molars, as long as they have permission slips and no decay. This needs to be done with a dentist to rule out caries first, and then they walk over to you for the sealants. It can be done in a library or gym, but is much easier at an office. All the second graders can get a "ticket" for a Saturday Clinic and you can get as many volunteers from the community as possible. The goal is fun, a little education, and an intro to the fact that dental offices aren't as scary as they previously thought (for both the kids and the parents). If you are lucky enough to have two dentists on board, one could restore the decay found as well. Having fun treats to hand out to the kids and a fantastic spread of donated baked goods for the staff make it a day you'll never forget. Take lots of pictures, have good coffee brewing and invite your local paper to come!

How to get your whole office involved

If you are lucky enough to work for someone who already has a "giving back" day, then kudos to you and your office! If you don't, why not suggest it at the next office meeting. I know it can be a lot of work, but it always comes back ten-fold! The people you treat may not become regular patients, but they may tell their boss about your generosity. Maybe he and his family haven't been to the dentist in years because they've been so busy making money and grinding their teeth...oh no, he might need full-mouth restoration! Wouldn't that be terrible? You'll always get a spot in the paper for these days...free advertising! Why not add in a free FMX and initial exam for new patients that month? I'm sure they can sneak that in the article somewhere (I write for my local paper, so I know stuff).

Liability

If you are worried about this subject, don't be. Just treat kids under 18 and stick to prophys, fluoride treatments, sealants and primary extractions (depending on your state laws). You do not have to follow up on the people you see, or finish their treatment needs. If your boss tells you that's why he doesn't want to get involved, call him out. It may take him out of his comfort zone and therefore require your persistence.

When I worked for Dr. Ash, she took our office manager (and my friend) Anita, 3 church volunteers and me down to Biloxi, MO one year after hurricane Katrina. We hauled a trailer full of donations from offices all around the Ann Arbor area, but Dr. Ash supplied most of it. We spent a week helping people from the community, so Samaritan's Purse was more than happy to give us room and board. They are easy to find in the face of natural disaster. They are usually neck and neck with the Red Cross to see who can set up shop first.

We saw over 100 people in four days. Almost all of them needed antibiotics and surgical extractions. Some had abscesses for a year because they were scheduled for a root canal or extraction the day the storm hit! Now Dr. Ash (a prosthodontist) is a petite woman that wears stilettos to work every day, and hadn't done this in years, but boy did she come through for these people. I stood in awe many times. What's more interesting is that her assistant was a 16 year old boy from her church who had never done any of this type of work before! The four of us put our faith in God that we could help as many people as possible and then spent our last day there doing demolition on someone's home so we could round out our experience. I will never forget the genuine gratitude these people exuded through their toothless smiles. You don't have to drive that far to make a difference, just open your front door.

Chapter 8~Going "GREEN"

"Waste not, want not"

Thinking of your impact on the environment

I added this chapter after starting the book because of my growing awareness for all that is wasted and unnatural. All I want to do is encourage you to make this a topic you promise yourself to learn more about in the coming year. Pay attention to what you throw away. Try to make more trips to Goodwill or the Salvation Army, and check out some re-sale shops for bargains and treasures. That's my favorite way of "recycling."

I've been green cleaning for the past year at home at would encourage all of you to start! It's easier than you think. All I use is baking soda, vinegar, and essential oils. You can find an array of recipes online at www.cleaning-green.net. If you happen to partake in the cleaning of your office, mention your new inexpensive way of cleaning to your boss. They won't make a fuss if it saves them money *and* works.

Transfer your home ways to the office

This is the easiest way to bring up recycling at your next office meeting. Just ask if you can do whatever you are currently doing at home, at work...no matter how big or small a part you play in the save the earth show. The easiest way I found to keep plastic garbage bags out of landfills is to dump each operatory garbage (sans bag) in the big bag in sterilization or the lab and take only that out at night. That keeps 4-10 smaller bags from hitting the landfill per day! Replace when needed.

Another way is to put a couple of plastic storage containers out (ours are in the entry way) and label them *plastic* and *paper*, they will fill up faster than you think! Check the bottom for the recycle triangle. The only effort is hauling them home and taking care of them when you take care of your own stuff. If you're not already going green at home because you're not sure if your waste company takes it, call and ask. They may charge you an extra $5 per month, so if you're that cheap you can haul it yourself. Go to www.recyclemore.org for collection sites in your area. It is work, but it's such a rewarding feeling when you cut down the amount of trash you put out each week by 50-80%. We sometimes fill up the plastic container in one day at work! Just be sure to rinse the chemicals out well before you send them home in Susie's new SUV, I speak from experience and the smell lingered for weeks!

What don't you need to treat patients

effectively and keep yourself safe?

This is a hard question to raise because of infection control, but I'll do it anyway. Back in the early 90's the dental supply companies came up with plastic covers for everything but your patients face! And they're bringing in major bucks because of it. I know it does cut down on the number of contaminated surfaces when you're sterilizing for the next patient, but do we really need all of it? OSHA recommends that we wipe twice whether something is covered or not, so can you cut down on one or two products that regularly are on auto order? Can you look for products that are made of something other than plastic? I know this may get shot down by your boss, but look at the cost of buying all this disposable stuff as well. With the economy the way it is, he or she may be thrilled that you've come up with a way of cutting supply costs and you can be thrilled with yourself for saving a small piece of your world (or landfill)! Also, be cautious when throwing a stack of 2x2's on every tray. Only put out what you truly think you will use.

Summary

Ways to pass on what you know

Undoubtedly there are some of you upset right now that the book is over and I didn't cover a topic as essential to your hygiene life as coffee is to mine. So, like I said in the Forward, maybe you should write your own book...I'd love to read it! This is in no way intended to be a full or expert opinion on all things dental hygiene. It's the opposite of that entirely. This is an "R" rated sneak-peak into the inner workings of my dental soul that have kept me going successfully for the duration of my career. It's the book I was unable to find when I started working as the only hygienist at an office, fresh out of school. The other reason I wrote this book was because I've been entertaining the idea of going back to school for Healthcare Administration and I didn't want all I've learned to slip away without sharing it...to literally anyone who cares to read about it. And please, if you do nothing else *new* after reading this, promise me you will find one rough spot to go back and scale while feeling with your floss at the end of the appointment. Remember, we *all* leave stuff behind...hopefully it's a smile or a kind word instead of calculus :o)

Tidbits you may not have been told in school

- Polish with course paste, then hand scale, then polish with fine paste for stain removal.
- Use the syringe cap to put a cotton tip applicator dipped in topical, and then it won't get all over.
- You can infiltrate with Articaine on the mandible. I haven't given a block in years!
- Three good ways to up production are to look for patients due for an FMX or PANX, spot scale and root plane even one pocket in need,

and to make sure anyone with multiple pockets over 4mm are on a 4 month recall. Those who build calculus quickly as well. A quicker recall is not just for those who have had periodontal treatment; it can be for those trying to avoid it as well. And it is usually at your discretion to suggest it.

- Give the patient choices whenever possible. It is their mouth and they will appreciate you saying, "If it was my mouth, I would do X, but you can also choose Y."

- Check for left over calculus while flossing after polishing!!! If you go nice and slow, wrapping well, you are likely to feel *something* you left behind. In fact, the better a hygienist is, the more often she catches herself!

- Check with your boss, but most offices do not take BWX while patients are in orthodontics.

- There are a number of new lasers on the market. They work on cold sores, tissue retraction and troughing for crowns, and some are even being used by hygienists to sterilize pockets in conjunction with perio treatment. Check with your boss to see if he has done any research. I watched an 11 mm pocket go to a 4mm pocket after one month of healing! This current generation of lasers is truly awesome. We may not even fully know all they can do. Look into it if you haven't already!

- Keep a list in your room of those patients that say they will "call when they have their schedule in front of them" to schedule restorative treatment. When you have down time, get it out. The hygienist calling them sometimes makes them think twice about putting it off.

- When you have a super sensitive patient, try applying desensitizer or MI Paste *before* scaling. Works wonders for me and I do not need to numb as many people up anymore.

- Invisalign is amazing. Another thing to suggest to your boss if you haven't looked into it. It has helped our production greatly and tons of patients who would've never considered traditional braces now have uncrowded, easy to clean teeth and gorgeous smiles. Gets the topic of *Full Mouth Restoration* going as well, and your boss will love that idea—cha ching!

- Send a nice "we miss you" letter when phone calls aren't working and it has been more than two years since a patient has been in for a prophy.

Pay it forward

If you enjoyed this honest perspective, please pass it along to another member of your staff. I've attempted to write in a way that would be enjoyed by the entire office. And also, if you made it all the way to the end (I rarely finish a book), could you promise to do one thing today that makes your world a better place? Pray for peace, visit an elderly neighbor, call your mom, or whatever! Just make giving an important part of each day. You'll soon find that you get more out of it than the person you give to anyway. Don't worry--the assistants will still let you keep your "Prima Donna" title for awhile. I just happen to prefer "Perio Princess" instead :o)

Thank you to:

Kelly Sweet/back cover photo www.kellysweet.com

Allison Bower/make-up www.allisonbower.com

CPSIA information can be obtained at www.ICGtesting.com
Printed in the USA
LVOW011954230513

335267LV00021B/596/P

9 781453 661963